# Non Scale Victories

## CELEBRATE WHAT YOU GAIN
## BECAUSE YOU LOST

# NSV

THIS WEEK:

- ○ MONDAY

- ○ TUESDAY

- ○ WEDNESDAY

- ○ THURSDAY

- ○ FRIDAY

- ○ SATURDAY / SUNDAY

# NON SCALE VICTORIES

# NSV

THIS WEEK:

- ○ MONDAY

- ○ TUESDAY

- ○ WEDNESDAY

- ○ THURSDAY

- ○ FRIDAY

- ○ SATURDAY / SUNDAY

# NON SCALE VICTORIES

# NSV

THIS WEEK:

- ○ MONDAY

- ○ TUESDAY

- ○ WEDNESDAY

- ○ THURSDAY

- ○ FRIDAY

- ○ SATURDAY / SUNDAY

# NON SCALE VICTORIES

# NSV



○ MONDAY

○ TUESDAY

○ WEDNESDAY

○ THURSDAY

○ FRIDAY

○ SATURDAY / SUNDAY

# NON SCALE VICTORIES

# NSV

THIS WEEK:

---

- ○ MONDAY

---

- ○ TUESDAY

---

- ○ WEDNESDAY

---

- ○ THURSDAY

---

- ○ FRIDAY

---

- ○ SATURDAY / SUNDAY

---

# NON SCALE VICTORIES

# NSV

THIS WEEK:

- ○ MONDAY

- ○ TUESDAY

- ○ WEDNESDAY

- ○ THURSDAY

- ○ FRIDAY

- ○ SATURDAY / SUNDAY

# NON SCALE VICTORIES

# NSV

THIS WEEK:

---

○ MONDAY

---

○ TUESDAY

---

○ WEDNESDAY

---

○ THURSDAY

---

○ FRIDAY

---

○ SATURDAY / SUNDAY

---

# NON SCALE VICTORIES

# NSV

THIS WEEK:

- ○ MONDAY

- ○ TUESDAY

- ○ WEDNESDAY

- ○ THURSDAY

- ○ FRIDAY

- ○ SATURDAY / SUNDAY

# NON SCALE VICTORIES

# NSV

THIS WEEK:

○ MONDAY

○ TUESDAY

○ WEDNESDAY

○ THURSDAY

○ FRIDAY

○ SATURDAY / SUNDAY

# NON SCALE VICTORIES

# NSV

THIS WEEK:

- ○ MONDAY

- ○ TUESDAY

- ○ WEDNESDAY

- ○ THURSDAY

- ○ FRIDAY

- ○ SATURDAY / SUNDAY

# NON SCALE VICTORIES

# NSV



- MONDAY

- TUESDAY

- WEDNESDAY

- THURSDAY

- FRIDAY

- SATURDAY / SUNDAY

# NON SCALE VICTORIES

# NSV

THIS WEEK:

- ○ MONDAY

- ○ TUESDAY

- ○ WEDNESDAY

- ○ THURSDAY

- ○ FRIDAY

- ○ SATURDAY / SUNDAY

# NON SCALE VICTORIES

# NSV

THIS WEEK:

○ MONDAY

○ TUESDAY

○ WEDNESDAY

○ THURSDAY

○ FRIDAY

○ SATURDAY / SUNDAY

# NON SCALE VICTORIES

# NSV

THIS WEEK:

- ○ MONDAY

- ○ TUESDAY

- ○ WEDNESDAY

- ○ THURSDAY

- ○ FRIDAY

- ○ SATURDAY / SUNDAY

# NON SCALE VICTORIES

# NSV

THIS WEEK:

- ○ MONDAY

- ○ TUESDAY

- ○ WEDNESDAY

- ○ THURSDAY

- ○ FRIDAY

- ○ SATURDAY / SUNDAY

# NON SCALE VICTORIES

# NSV

THIS WEEK:

---

- ○ MONDAY

---

- ○ TUESDAY

---

- ○ WEDNESDAY

---

- ○ THURSDAY

---

- ○ FRIDAY

---

- ○ SATURDAY / SUNDAY

---

# NON SCALE VICTORIES

# NSV



○ MONDAY

○ TUESDAY

○ WEDNESDAY

○ THURSDAY

○ FRIDAY

○ SATURDAY / SUNDAY

# NON SCALE VICTORIES

# NSV

THIS WEEK:

---

○ MONDAY

---

○ TUESDAY

---

○ WEDNESDAY

---

○ THURSDAY

---

○ FRIDAY

---

○ SATURDAY / SUNDAY

---

# NON SCALE VICTORIES

# NSV

THIS WEEK:

---

○ MONDAY

---

○ TUESDAY

---

○ WEDNESDAY

---

○ THURSDAY

---

○ FRIDAY

---

○ SATURDAY / SUNDAY

---

# NON SCALE VICTORIES

# NSV

THIS WEEK:

- ○ MONDAY

- ○ TUESDAY

- ○ WEDNESDAY

- ○ THURSDAY

- ○ FRIDAY

- ○ SATURDAY / SUNDAY

# NON SCALE VICTORIES

# NSV



○ MONDAY

○ TUESDAY

○ WEDNESDAY

○ THURSDAY

○ FRIDAY

○ SATURDAY / SUNDAY

# NON SCALE VICTORIES

# NSV

THIS WEEK:

○ MONDAY

○ TUESDAY

○ WEDNESDAY

○ THURSDAY

○ FRIDAY

○ SATURDAY / SUNDAY

# NON SCALE VICTORIES

# NSV

THIS WEEK:

- ○ MONDAY

- ○ TUESDAY

- ○ WEDNESDAY

- ○ THURSDAY

- ○ FRIDAY

- ○ SATURDAY / SUNDAY

# NON SCALE VICTORIES

# NSV

THIS WEEK:

- ○ MONDAY

- ○ TUESDAY

- ○ WEDNESDAY

- ○ THURSDAY

- ○ FRIDAY

- ○ SATURDAY / SUNDAY

# NON SCALE VICTORIES

# NSV

THIS WEEK:

- ○ MONDAY

- ○ TUESDAY

- ○ WEDNESDAY

- ○ THURSDAY

- ○ FRIDAY

- ○ SATURDAY / SUNDAY

# NON SCALE VICTORIES

# NSV

THIS WEEK:

- ○ MONDAY

- ○ TUESDAY

- ○ WEDNESDAY

- ○ THURSDAY

- ○ FRIDAY

- ○ SATURDAY / SUNDAY

# NON SCALE VICTORIES

# NSV

THIS WEEK:

- ○ MONDAY

- ○ TUESDAY

- ○ WEDNESDAY

- ○ THURSDAY

- ○ FRIDAY

- ○ SATURDAY / SUNDAY

# NON SCALE VICTORIES

# NSV



- ○ MONDAY

- ○ TUESDAY

- ○ WEDNESDAY

- ○ THURSDAY

- ○ FRIDAY

- ○ SATURDAY / SUNDAY

# NON SCALE VICTORIES

# NSV

THIS WEEK:

---

- ○ MONDAY

---

- ○ TUESDAY

---

- ○ WEDNESDAY

---

- ○ THURSDAY

---

- ○ FRIDAY

---

- ○ SATURDAY / SUNDAY

---

# NON SCALE VICTORIES

# NSV

THIS WEEK:

- ○ MONDAY

- ○ TUESDAY

- ○ WEDNESDAY

- ○ THURSDAY

- ○ FRIDAY

- ○ SATURDAY / SUNDAY

# NON SCALE VICTORIES

# NSV

THIS WEEK:

- ○ MONDAY

- ○ TUESDAY

- ○ WEDNESDAY

- ○ THURSDAY

- ○ FRIDAY

- ○ SATURDAY / SUNDAY

# NON SCALE VICTORIES

# NSV

THIS WEEK:

- ○ MONDAY

- ○ TUESDAY

- ○ WEDNESDAY

- ○ THURSDAY

- ○ FRIDAY

- ○ SATURDAY / SUNDAY

# NON SCALE VICTORIES

# NSV

THIS WEEK:

○ MONDAY

○ TUESDAY

○ WEDNESDAY

○ THURSDAY

○ FRIDAY

○ SATURDAY / SUNDAY

# NON SCALE VICTORIES

# NSV



- ○ MONDAY

- ○ TUESDAY

- ○ WEDNESDAY

- ○ THURSDAY

- ○ FRIDAY

- ○ SATURDAY / SUNDAY

# NON SCALE VICTORIES

# NSV

THIS WEEK:

---

○ MONDAY

---

○ TUESDAY

---

○ WEDNESDAY

---

○ THURSDAY

---

○ FRIDAY

---

○ SATURDAY / SUNDAY

---

# NON SCALE VICTORIES

# NSV



- MONDAY

- TUESDAY

- WEDNESDAY

- THURSDAY

- FRIDAY

- SATURDAY / SUNDAY

# NON SCALE VICTORIES

# NSV

THIS WEEK:

- ○ MONDAY

---

- ○ TUESDAY

---

- ○ WEDNESDAY

---

- ○ THURSDAY

---

- ○ FRIDAY

---

- ○ SATURDAY / SUNDAY

# NON SCALE VICTORIES

# NSV

THIS WEEK:

- ○ MONDAY

- ○ TUESDAY

- ○ WEDNESDAY

- ○ THURSDAY

- ○ FRIDAY

- ○ SATURDAY / SUNDAY

# NON SCALE VICTORIES

# NSV

THIS WEEK:

○ MONDAY

○ TUESDAY

○ WEDNESDAY

○ THURSDAY

○ FRIDAY

○ SATURDAY / SUNDAY

# NON SCALE VICTORIES

# NSV

THIS WEEK:

---

○ MONDAY

---

○ TUESDAY

---

○ WEDNESDAY

---

○ THURSDAY

---

○ FRIDAY

---

○ SATURDAY / SUNDAY

---

# NON SCALE VICTORIES

# NSV



○ MONDAY

○ TUESDAY

○ WEDNESDAY

○ THURSDAY

○ FRIDAY

○ SATURDAY / SUNDAY

# NON SCALE VICTORIES

# NSV

THIS WEEK:

- ○ MONDAY

- ○ TUESDAY

- ○ WEDNESDAY

- ○ THURSDAY

- ○ FRIDAY

- ○ SATURDAY / SUNDAY

# NON SCALE VICTORIES

# NSV

THIS WEEK:

- ○ MONDAY

- ○ TUESDAY

- ○ WEDNESDAY

- ○ THURSDAY

- ○ FRIDAY

- ○ SATURDAY / SUNDAY

# NON SCALE VICTORIES

# NSV



- MONDAY
- TUESDAY
- WEDNESDAY
- THURSDAY
- FRIDAY
- SATURDAY / SUNDAY

# NON SCALE VICTORIES

# NSV

THIS WEEK:

- ○ MONDAY

- ○ TUESDAY

- ○ WEDNESDAY

- ○ THURSDAY

- ○ FRIDAY

- ○ SATURDAY / SUNDAY

# NON SCALE VICTORIES

# NSV

THIS WEEK:

- ○ MONDAY

- ○ TUESDAY

- ○ WEDNESDAY

- ○ THURSDAY

- ○ FRIDAY

- ○ SATURDAY / SUNDAY

# NON SCALE VICTORIES

# NSV

THIS WEEK:

---

○ MONDAY

---

○ TUESDAY

---

○ WEDNESDAY

---

○ THURSDAY

---

○ FRIDAY

---

○ SATURDAY / SUNDAY

---

# NON SCALE VICTORIES

# NSV



○ MONDAY

○ TUESDAY

○ WEDNESDAY

○ THURSDAY

○ FRIDAY

○ SATURDAY / SUNDAY

# NON SCALE VICTORIES

# NSV

THIS WEEK:

- ○ MONDAY

- ○ TUESDAY

- ○ WEDNESDAY

- ○ THURSDAY

- ○ FRIDAY

- ○ SATURDAY / SUNDAY

# NON SCALE VICTORIES

# NSV

THIS WEEK:

- ○ MONDAY

- ○ TUESDAY

- ○ WEDNESDAY

- ○ THURSDAY

- ○ FRIDAY

- ○ SATURDAY / SUNDAY

# NON SCALE VICTORIES

# NSV

THIS WEEK:

- ○ MONDAY

- ○ TUESDAY

- ○ WEDNESDAY

- ○ THURSDAY

- ○ FRIDAY

- ○ SATURDAY / SUNDAY

# NON SCALE VICTORIES

# NSV

THIS WEEK:

- ○ MONDAY

- ○ TUESDAY

- ○ WEDNESDAY

- ○ THURSDAY

- ○ FRIDAY

- ○ SATURDAY / SUNDAY

# NON SCALE VICTORIES

On To More

Victories

www.ingramcontent.com/pod-product-compliance
Lightning Source LLC
Chambersburg PA
CBHW081726250726
48657CB00010B/3156